Power of Pilates

Achieving Nutritional and Physical Balance

Table of Contents

Chapter 1. Introduction

Step into the world of transformation in our special report, "The Power of Pilates: Achieving Nutritional and Physical Balance." This compelling report dives deep into the fascinating fusion of Pilates and nutrition, shedding light on how this power-duo can propel individuals to greater heights of health and fitness. Fun, engaging, and perfect for those yearning to move towards a more balanced lifestyle, it's filled with practical advice, expert insights, and real-life success stories. This fresh perspective will enrich you with knowledge, inspire your journey, and offer a roadmap to a healthier you. So, why wait? Elevate your well-being and leap into an enriching journey of balance, strength, and flexibility. Get your hands on this exclusive report now, and let's start transforming together!

Chapter 2. Unveiling the Power of Pilates

Pilates is far more than simply another exercise routine; it's a comprehensive system designed to engage the body and mind in concert, resulting in enhanced physical strength, flexibility, and mental clarity. Pioneered by Joseph Pilates in the early twentieth century, Pilates pushes boundaries beyond traditional workout regimes, fostering an elevation of mind-body awareness that inspires overall wellbeing.

2.1. Defining Pilates

Pilates is a method of exercise that consists of low-impact flexibility, muscular strength and endurance movements. Named after its founder, Joseph Pilates, it emphasizes the use of the mind to control muscles, focusing attention on core postural muscles that help keep the body balanced and provide support for the spine. In this context, 'core' refers primarily to the abdomen, lower back, hips and buttocks.

Pilates classes typically take 45 minutes to an hour and are performed on a mat or on specialized equipment. It is an adaptable exercise regime, suitable for all age groups and fitness levels, focusing on alignment, breathing, developing a strong core, and improving balance and coordination.

2.2. Historical Overview

Joseph Pilates was born in Germany in 1883. He was a sickly child, suffering from rickets, asthma and rheumatic fever. Determined to overcome his physical ailments, he began to study anatomy and exercise, practicing various disciplines such as gymnastics, bodybuilding, and martial arts.

By World War I, Pilates had developed a system of exercises and innovative equipment to assist detainees in rehabilitating and maintaining their health while being held in internment camps. Post-war, he migrated to the United States and opened his own studio in New York City in 1926, offering his comprehensive method of physical and mental conditioning, which he called 'contrology.'

Importantly, Pilates was decades ahead of his time in understanding that physical health, mental wellbeing, proper breathing, and adequate sleep are interdependent facets of overall health.

2.3. Principles of Pilates

There are six key principles central to Pilates:

1. **Concentration**: Pilates requires mental focus to maintain correct form.

2. **Control**: Every movement should be performed with control to avoid injury and produce positive results.

3. **Centering**: Activities are focused around the 'center' or 'powerhouse' of the torso.

4. **Flow**: There is a flowing grace to each movement, with one activity flowing smoothly into the next.

5. **Precision**: Each movement is performed precisely to get the most benefit, and to eliminate unproductive energy use.

6. **Breathing**: Joseph Pilates promoted a method of breathing with intent, inspiring a cleansing of the body and mind.

2.4. The Power of Pilates

Pilates has emerged as one of the best ways to engage your body and mind synchronously, leading to multiple health benefits:

1. **Improves Flexibility**: Regular practice improves flexibility, with exercises that lengthen muscles and increase range of motion.

2. **Builds Strength**: Pilates exercises focus on strengthening the body's 'core' or 'powerhouse' (torso). But that doesn't mean the other body parts don't get a workout— they do.

3. **Develops Control and Stability**: Pilates encourages better posture, balance, and body mechanics, which are crucial for daily activities, reducing the chance of injury.

4. **Promotes Mind-Body Awareness**: With its emphasis on mindful movement, Pilates enhances body awareness. Practitioners find themselves moving more gracefully and with improved ease in daily life.

5. **Boosts Mental Health**: Its focus on controlled breathing and quality, not quantity, of movement, Pilates has a meditative quality that fosters stress relief and promotes mental wellbeing.

2.5. Common Pilates Movements

There are over 500 exercises in the traditional Pilates repertoire, with modifications and variations available to accommodate all fitness levels, including:

1. **The Hundred**: This is a warm-up exercise that gets your body ready for the regimen. It focuses on core strength and rhythmic breathing.

2. **The Roll Up**: This is a slow, deliberate movement that stretches the spine and the back muscles, and tests your core strength.

3. **The Bridge**: This exercise targets your powerhouse area and works your buttocks, hips, and lower back.

4. **The Swan**: This exercise strengthens the back of your body and improves the flexibility of your spine.

5. **The Leg Pull**: This movement works your abs and tests your

balance.

To conclude, Pilates is a potent tool in the search for improved fitness and wellbeing. With its focus on core strength, flexibility, and mindfulness, Pilates offers a holistic approach to personal health, from enhancing muscle tone to fostering mental acuity. The positive impact spills over into everyday activity, improving posture, reducing the risk of injury, and boosting confidence. With committed practice, Pilates can be transformative in helping individuals achieve balance in their body and a buoyant sense of wellbeing in their life.

Chapter 3. Aligning Body and Mind: The Core Principle

A truly holistic approach to health acknowledges the inextricable link that exists between our physical bodies and our mental state. Pilates, a practice steeped in the principles of concentration, control, centering, flow, precision, and breathing, offers a profound way to synchronise both these aspects of our being. By incorporating sound nutritional habits alongside Pilates, we foster an environment conducive to the seamless alignment of mind and body.

3.1. The Symbiotic Relationship of Mind and Body

Scientific research increasingly supports the symbiotic relationship between our mental and physical health. Studies have shown that stress and negative emotions can negatively influence physical health, exacerbating ailments and suppressing our immune system. Conversely, physical illnesses often produce psychological symptoms. Therefore, achieving a healthy mind-body alignment, as taught in Pilates alongside sound nutritional practices, can greatly enhance our overall well-being.

Pilates' concept of centering relates directly to this principle. Coined by Joseph Pilates as the "powerhouse" of the body, the center involves a group of muscles in the middle of the body—encompassing the lower back, abdomen, hips, and buttocks. Pilates exercises commence from this core and flow outward to the extremities, analogous to the way our thoughts and emotions (originating from the brain) ripple out to affect our body.

3.2. Pilates: A Tool for Body-Mind Integration

By drawing our attention towards movement and breath, Pilates exercises cultivate an enhanced body awareness. This refined perception allows us to notice and correct unhealthy movement patterns, improve posture, and decrease physical tension.

In Pilates, breath is viewed as the life force that energizes the body and mind. Joseph Pilates strongly emphasized using precise, controlled breathwork to oxygenate the blood and to activate deep abdominal and pelvic floor muscles—essential for developing core strength and stability.

Mastering the Pilates breathing technique—inhale through the nose to prepare, then exhale through the mouth during the most effortful part of an exercise—concentrates the mind and helps to coordinate movement. This method, while improving physical performance, also cultivates mindfulness, a mental state achieved by focusing awareness on the present moment.

Research indicates that mindfulness plays a critical role in mental health—reducing stress, anxiety, and depression. Depending on how it is practiced, Pilates can practically serve as a moving meditation, encouraging practitioners to be fully present – deepening the mind-body connection.

3.3. Nutrition: The Physical Basis of Mental Well-being

It's no secret that the foods we consume significantly affect our physical health. However, emerging research also indicates a strong link between diet and mental well-being. This correlation is so strong that an entirely new field, nutritional psychiatry, has emerged.

Certain nutrients are important for the production of neurotransmitters—chemical messengers that contribute to our mood and cognitive function. For example, omega-3 fatty acids, found abundantly in fish, walnuts, and chia seeds, are vital for brain health and have been linked to a reduced risk of depressive disorders. Likewise, carbohydrates with a low glycemic index, like whole grains, help maintain stable blood sugar levels—thus providing the brain with a steady energy supply and combating mood swings.

Nutrition and hydration are equally crucial in physical performance, including Pilates practice. Well-nourished bodies have the energy necessary for effective Pilates sessions and proper hydration supports muscle function, flexibility, and concentration.

3.4. Aligning Nutrition and Pilates: A Balanced Blueprint

It's important to create a nutrition plan that supports your Pilates regimen and other life demands, and vice versa. A balanced, nutrient-rich diet—consisting of lean proteins, complex carbohydrates, healthy fats, and plenty of fruits and vegetables—provides the necessary fuel for your body while promoting mental clarity.

Consider eating a small, balanced meal or snack 1-2 hours before your Pilates class to ensure you have enough energy for the workout. A combination of lean protein and complex carbohydrates could be an excellent choice. Following your workout, focus on replenishing your energy stores and repairing your muscles, for example, a smoothie with protein, fruits and some healthy fat.

3.5. The Real-Life Impact

The combination of Pilates and nutritional focus brings about physical transformations—increased strength and flexibility, improved posture, more efficient movement, and often, weight loss. In addition, practitioners often report improved concentration, better stress management, and an increased sense of peace and satisfaction.

A daily Pilates practice grounded in sound nutritional habits enhances the connection between mind and body. Over time, this internal balance and harmony become integrated into our everyday lives, beyond the classroom. Pilates practitioners often find they're not only physically stronger and more flexible, but more mindful during daily tasks and more attuned to their bodies' nutritional needs.

In conclusion, a consistent Pilates routine, enhanced by a solid nutritional plan, strengthens the body, nourishes the mind, and lays a solid framework for a truly balanced lifestyle, authentic well-being, and optimal health. Incorporating these practices into your life can be transformative, regardless of age, fitness level, or health status.

Chapter 4. Nutritional Insights: Fuelling Your Pilates Practice

Pilates has gained considerable acclaim as a regimen for enhancing strength, flexibility, balance, and overall physical fitness. Still, it's crucial not to lose sight that feeding your body properly is equally as vital for yielding optimum results. When it comes to this, understanding good nutrition is key.

4.1. The Importance of Nutrition in Pilates

What we consume fuels our bodies for day-to-day activities and workouts. An appropriate and balanced diet is a prerequisite for maintaining the energy levels required during Pilates sessions. Your energy, stamina, fat loss, and muscle gain are highly dependent on what you eat and when you eat.

Your body requires a specific set of macro and micronutrients to function appropriately, and each nutrient plays a definitive role in maintaining optimal health and enabling performance. The balance between proteins, carbohydrates, and fats, along with adequate hydration, can significantly impact your Pilates performance.

4.2. Understanding Macronutrients

When we talk about macronutrients, we are referring to proteins, carbohydrates, and fats. Each of these plays an essential role in body functioning and should be incorporated into our diets in the correct ratios.

Proteins are the building blocks of muscles. They assist in repairing and building muscle tissues, especially after a rigorous Pilates session. Foods rich in proteins include lean meats, fish, dairy products, beans, and nuts.

Carbohydrates are the primary energy source for our bodies. They fuel muscles during exercises, whether it's a Pilates class, a jog, or a strength training session. Opt for complex carbohydrates like whole grains, vegetables, fruits, and legumes, as they offer sustained energy release.

Fats are also an important part of a healthy diet. They act as a secondary source of energy, aid in the absorption of fat-soluble vitamins, and are critical for cell functioning. Favor unsaturated fats found in avocados, fish, nuts, and olive oil, and limit the intake of saturated and trans fats.

4.3. How to Fuel Before, During, and After Pilates

To ensure sufficient energy during your Pilates practice, timing your meals and understanding the type of nutrients required is vital.

Before a Session: It's generally advisable to consume a balanced meal containing proteins and carbohydrates 2-3 hours before working out. This provides ample energy and avoids any digestive discomfort during the session. For those who prefer early morning classes, a quick snack that includes a small portion of simple carbohydrates and proteins will suffice.

During a Session: Hydration is crucial. Sip water during your Pilates routine to replenish lost fluids and avoid dehydration.

After a Session: Post-Pilates nutrition aims to replenish glycogen stores and repair muscle tissue. Having a meal or snack containing proteins and carbohydrates within 45 minutes after the session can help achieve this.

4.4. The Role of Micronutrients

Vitamins and minerals (micronutrients) also play a pivotal role in maintaining optimal health and enhancing Pilates performance. They are essential for a myriad of bodily functions, including energy production, bone health, immunity, and wound healing.

Vitamin D and calcium are vital for bone health and muscle function. Iron helps in energy production and oxygen transport. Antioxidants like vitamins C, E, and selenium combat oxidative stress occurring during workouts. A balanced diet incorporating a variety of fruits, vegetables, whole grains, lean proteins, and healthy fats should provide these micronutrients. If not, supplements may be considered after consulting a healthcare professional.

4.5. Understanding Hydration

During a Pilates session, your body loses water through sweat. Staying hydrated is critical for maintaining body temperature, transporting nutrients and oxygen to cells, and getting rid of body wastes. Ensure you start your Pilates session well-hydrated, preferably sip water during the session, and definitely drink fluids after working out to replenish lost fluids.

Incorporating these nutritional insights into your Pilates practice can significantly improve performance, promoting muscle growth and recovery, and optimizing energy utilization. Remember, each individual is different, and these principles should be adapted according to personal needs, preferences, and goals. Well-balanced nutrition goes hand-in-hand with Pilates for reaching health and fitness goals.

Chapter 5. Pilates 101: A Comprehensive Guide for Beginners

As a holistic approach to health and wellness, Pilates combines strength, balance, flexibility, and mindfulness. Combining a variety of exercises that are both low-impact and adaptable, it is suitable for individuals of all fitness levels. Let's explore this journey of understanding Pilates from its basics.

5.1. What Is Pilates?

Pilates is a physical fitness system pioneered by Joseph Pilates in the early 20th century. At its core, Pilates aims to create a balance between the mind and body, focusing on strength, flexibility, and overall body awareness. The system is renowned for its ability to improve posture, muscle tone, balance and joint mobility, often making it a go-to exercise regimen for rehabilitation and prevention of musculoskeletal injuries.

5.2. Principles of Pilates

Essential to any Pilates workout, six core principles form the basis of every movement:

1. Centering: The physical focus of your workout is the center of the body, often defined as the area between the ribs and the pubic bone. This focus helps to stabilize your torso and control your movements.

2. Concentration: Every exercise demands your focus on each movement, thereby connecting the mind to the body.

3. Control: Joseph Pilates stressed meticulous control over each movement, preferring fewer, precise movements over uncontrolled repetitions.

4. Precision: The quality of each movement is more important than the quantity or speed, requiring conscientious execution of each position.

5. Breath: Proper breathe control is crucial in Pilates; uniform and coordinated breathing should complement each action.

6. Flow: Movements in Pilates should be fluid, connecting each pose with grace and with the rhythm of one's breath.

5.3. Essential Pilates Positions for Beginners

To get started with Pilates, familiarize yourself with these basic exercises:

1. The Hundred: A classic Pilates warm-up exercise that challenges your abdominal muscles and your breathing coordination.

2. Pilates Roll Up: A full sit-up that promotes spinal articulation and targets your core muscles.

3. Single Leg Circles: This helps to enhance mobility in the hips and strengthens the core.

4. The Bridge: Great for toning the glutes, hamstrings and core while also stretching the chest and spine.

5. Criss Cross: This exercise is designed to engage the oblique muscles and helps promote upper body rotation and flexibility.

5.4. Links Between Pilates and Nutrition

Integrating Pilates with nutrition inevitably means not just working on the outside physique but also nurturing the body from within. The emphasis should be on consuming a well-rounded diet filled with a variety of nutrient-dense foods that enhance your Pilates practice and optimize recovery post-workout. Prioritize quality protein to assist muscle repair and growth, complex carbohydrates for sustained energy, and plenty of fruits and vegetables for their vast array of health-promoting micronutrients and antioxidants.

5.5. Making Pilates Part of Your Daily Routine

While starting with Pilates, it's not necessary to devote hours each day; even 10 to 15 minutes can make a difference. Gradually increase the time dedicating about 3-4 days a week to see real improvements.

Remember, consistency matters more than the duration of each workout. And as you progress, increase the number and complexity of the poses, challenging your body in new ways. Incorporate your learnings from the Pilates practice into your everyday life, focusing on maintaining correct postures and using your body's core to support movements.

5.6. Final Thoughts

Begin your journey to superior health with a humble understanding of Pilates' principles, mastering basic exercises, and embracing nutritious eating habits. Regular practice of Pilates, associated with balanced nutrition, can help you enhance strength, improve flexibility, and develop a keen mindfulness about your body. With patience and persistence, the art and science of Pilates can guide you to a more balanced and healthy lifestyle.

That said, remember, everyone's body is unique, and what may work for one may not work for another. Always listen to your body and seek professional advice if intending to make significant changes to your exercise or nutrition regime.

Chapter 6. Inspirational Stories: Transformations through Pilates and Nutrition

Every journey begins somewhere. In the world of health transformation, every journey starts with one decision – the decision to improve, to change, to transform. This chapter houses stories of individuals who've embarked on this journey, finding in Pilates and nutrition, a tool of change powerful enough to transform their lives.

6.1. From Far and Wide: Elizabeth Cole's Journey to Transformation

Elizabeth Cole was a 32-year-old entrepreneur with a blossoming startup to manage. She found herself frequently stressed, juggling numerous responsibilities while skipping meals and exercise. Elizabeth noticed a growing lethargy taking hold, a persistent state of exhaustion that began affecting her work performance and overall well-being.

A chance encounter at a wellness seminar introduced her to the fusion of Pilates and nutrition. Intriguingly, it advocated not only for physical fitness but also nutritional balance, which spoke to her need for energy management and overall well-being.

Opting for a 60-minute Pilates session thrice a week, combined with a dietary overhaul planned by a certified nutritionist, Elizabeth embarked on her transformative journey. She found that the combination of nutritious food and energizing Pilates gave her the much-needed lift in her energy levels. Eight months into her new routine, not only had she increased her strength, flexibility, and muscle tone, but her energy levels were consistently high, leading to improved performance at work.

6.2. Zero to Hero: Tom Branson's Route to Redemption

Tom Branson was a 45-year-old office worker with a sedentary lifestyle that had led to obesity. He was lethargic, had low self-esteem and was pre-diabetic. Encouraged by his family, Tom decided to transform his life.

Tom turned to Pilates as his exercise of choice, having heard of its low impact on joints and inclusive nature for all body types. He also decided to consult a nutritionist to alter his diet. A personalized meal plan later, Tom was ready.

Daily Pilates sessions combined with a balanced diet full of lean proteins and vegetables brought visible transformations within months. Over the course of a year, Tom lost a total of 80 pounds, gained muscle definition, regained his self-esteem and energy, and reversed his pre-diabetes. Tom's story is a testament to how Pilates and nutrition can overhaul one's health completely.

6.3. Transformation against all odds: Olivia Harper's Tale

Olivia Harper, a classical ballet dancer, suffered a critical knee injury that threatened to end her career. Post-surgery, Olivia felt her strength and flexibility waning, causing desolation. Desperate for a solution, she turned to Pilates in an attempt to regain her strength.

Alongside focused Pilates, Olivia also paid attention to her nutrition, targeting muscle repair and strength. She increased her intake of protein, fruits, vegetables and complex carbohydrates, all while continuing her rehabilitation-focused Pilates exercises.

In two years, Olivia not only made a remarkable recovery but returned to her ballet practice stronger than ever. Her story stands as a beacon of hope, demonstrating the power of Pilates and nutrition even in the face of the direst circumstances.

6.4. The Blossom of Age: Mary Stone's Unlikely Transformation

Mary Stone was a 65-year-old grandmother who believed it was 'too late' to start a fitness regime. However, she yearned the agility to play with her grandkids without losing breath. Finally, she discovered Pilates, an exercise suitable for her age that wouldn't add unwanted stress to her joints.

In conjunction with Pilates, Mary also altered her diet, incorporating more vegetables, grains, lean proteins and fruits. Within months, Mary noticed newfound energy, lost considerable weight, and gained muscle strength. She successfully thwarted the 'too late' myth, showing that any age is a good age to start a healthful journey.

These transformation stories bring forward the trend of individuals achieving their health goals through Pilates and nutrition. Despite diverse backgrounds and varying challenges, the common thread among them was the decision to embrace change, nurtured by the nourishing alliance of Pilates and nutrition. They have proven that with consistency and dedication, transformation is within reach for everyone.

Chapter 7. The Science Behind Pilates and Nutritional Balance

Pilates, an exercise method designed to improve physical strength, flexibility, posture, and mental awareness, has found a profound synergy when paired with proper nutrition. Individually, they play crucial roles in health and wellness, but together, they form a formidable fusion that turns the dial on personal health and fitness.

7.1. The Underlying Principles of Pilates

Pilates fundamentally revolves around six key principles: centering, concentration, control, precision, breath, and flow. These principles act as the structure upon which the comprehensive Pilates method is built. From mat exercises to specific apparatus workouts, every Pilates move aims to embody these principles.

1. *Centering*: Every movement in Pilates is generated from the 'powerhouse,' an area roughly bound by the lower ribs and hips. This notion of centering goes beyond physical and taps into the emotional and spiritual aspects of wellness.

2. *Concentration*: Pilates demands focused attention and awareness. By concentrating on the body's movements, one can achieve heightened body awareness and more accurate execution of exercises.

3. *Control*: Rather than relying on momentum, Pilates emphasizes maintaining control throughout exercises. This level of control aids in injury prevention.

4. *Precision*: The effectiveness of Pilates lies in the precision of

movements. Each exercise is designed with intentional alignment and action.

5. *Breath*: Breathwork is integral to Pilates. It ensures that oxygen flows freely around the body, promoting better energy levels and creating a rhythmic pattern for the execution of exercises.

6. *Flow*: Pilates exercises are performed smoothly to maintain the fluidity and grace of movements, improving both physical conditioning and cognitive coordination.

7.2. Analyzing Pilates Benefits

Pilates offers a myriad of health benefits, making it a popular choice for fitness enthusiasts of all demographics. It's an especially beneficial practice for improving core strength, flexibility, posture, and balance, all of which are essential for maintaining functional movement and overall health.

1. *Improving Core Strength*: The exercises in Pilates are geared toward strengthening the core, improving stability and overall body strength.

2. *Increasing Flexibility*: Through the structured and repetitive movements, Pilates can help increase the flexibility and length of the muscles.

3. *Better Posture*: The focus on the core and the precision of movements can result in better posture. This can yield a multitude of health benefits like reducing the risk of back pain and improving respiratory health.

4. *Enhanced Balance and Coordination*: The balance fostered through Pilates can be significant in reducing the risk of falls, especially in the older population. Simultaneously, performing the exercises can help improve body awareness and coordination.

7.3. The Role of Nutrition in Fitness

While physical movement forms the basis of fitness, it is through nutrition that our bodies extract the energy to perform these activities. Proper nutrition forms the essential underpinning for not only maintaining health, but also optimizing physical performance. The body needs a variety of nutrients to function optimally: proteins for muscle repair and growth, carbohydrates for energy, fats for hormone production, vitamins, and minerals for various metabolic processes.

7.4. The Symbiosis of Pilates and Nutrition

When Pilates and nutrition are integrated, their potential health contributions are massively amplified. A robust nutritional plan can fuel the body for Pilates workouts, aid in recovery between sessions, and ensure the body secures maximum benefit from each training.

1. *Creating a Nutrient-Dense Eating Plan*: The essence of nutritional balance as a companion to Pilates is to consume a nutrient-dense diet. A diet packed with lean proteins, a variety of vegetables and fruits, whole grains, and healthy fats aids in muscle repair and development.

2. *Hydration*: Hydration is important to support the increased activity level during Pilates. Drinking water regularly helps in maintaining optimal body temperature, lubricating joints, and transporting nutrients for energy and health.

3. *Pairing Timing with Nutrient Needs*: Consuming the right nutrients at the right time is a crucial aspect to maximize the efficiency of Pilates workouts.

7.5. Pilates and Balanced Nutrition – A Road to Healthier Lifestyle

The integration of Pilates and a balanced nutritional diet can escalate the journey towards a healthier lifestyle. This fusion can be a significant step towards managing weight, reducing the risk of various diseases, having better mental health, and improving overall quality of life.

By placing equal importance on dedicated Pilates training and a balanced, nutrient-rich diet, individuals can promote their own holistic wellness, building not only physical resilience, but also fostering an attitude of mindfulness and inner peace. This all-around positive influence is why more people are being drawn towards Pilates and nutrition as their trusted companions on the road to a healthier lifestyle.

Chapter 8. Optimizing Your Routine: Building a Personalized Pilates and Nutrition Plan

In this journey towards personal transformation, it is essential to customize your Pilates regimen and nutritional plan according to your needs. Gaining a comprehensive understanding of the principles of Pilates and the role of nutritional balance will enable you to tap into a world of health, fitness, and inner harmony.

8.1. Understanding Your Body's Needs

Every person is different, and so are their needs. Knowing your body's requirements is crucial to creating an effective personalized Pilates and nutrition plan. Approaching this requires careful assessment of your current health status, fitness goals, dietary habits, and lifestyle factors.

Perform a physical inventory starting with your weight, muscle mass, body fat percentage, strength, flexibility, and other health indicators. This data can be collected using bioelectrical impedance devices, skinfold calipers, strength tests, and flexibility measures.

Next, reflect on your diet, including what you eat, how much you eat, and when you eat. Track your dietary patterns for several days to a week. Try to maintain a comprehensive approach, capturing everything – from whole meals to small bites, snacking trends, and drink consumption.

Goal-setting enhances the productivity of your routine. These could be a mix of long-term and short-term objectives focusing on weight loss, muscle toning, improving flexibility, increasing cardiovascular health, stress reduction, or dietary changes.

It's important to also pay heed to psycho-social factors. Understand the stressors and challenges in your life, as these could directly influence your diet and dedication to the Pilates program. This understanding will equip you to better cope with these variables and make well-rounded decisions for your health.

8.2. Designing Your Personalized Pilates Workout

Once you have a clear understanding of your requirements, goals, and lifestyle, you can structure your Pilates routine. It's recommended to start slow, with a greater emphasis on learning the right techniques correctly rather than doing as many exercises as possible.

Your Pilates routine should comprise the six fundamental Pilates principles: centering, control, flow, breath, precision, and concentration. Adapt these principles to your specific needs.

Start with basic exercises that target your core as it is the heart of all Pilates movements. Then, gradually introduce exercises which target other areas that align with your fitness goals.

Select an appropriate setting for your workout – be it a serene corner at home or a Pilates studio. Choose a time of the day when you can maintain regularity with minimum interruptions. Creating an environment that encourages mindfulness and concentration will amplify the benefits derived from Pilates practice.

You may choose to hire a skilled Pilates instructor for guidance, especially when you are just starting. Their expertise can help guide you through advanced exercises, monitor your progress, and make the required changes to your routine.

8.3. Crafting Your Personalized Nutrition Plan

Aligning Pilates-centric fitness goals with your food intake is imperative. Crafting a personalized nutrition plan isn't just about eating less or more – but eating right and balanced.

Begin by calculating your daily calorie intake requirements based on your physical composition and activity levels. BMR calculators and Harris-Benedict Equation are commonly used tools.

Ensure a well-balanced proportion of macronutrients for your daily consumption: proteins, carbohydrates, and fats. Proteins are a must for muscle building and repair, whole carbohydrates provide the necessary energy, while healthy fats support overall well-being.

Incorporate a good mix of micronutrients (vitamins, minerals). Introduce colorful fruits and vegetables, beans, nuts, seeds, lean meats, and whole grains in your diet. These consist of all the necessary nutrients and fibers required for your body.

Understanding the concepts of portion control and how to read nutrition labels on food packaging will empower you with your dietary choices.

Given the intensity of Pilates, pre and post-workout meals are critical. A balanced meal with protein, a bit of fat, and some complex carbs will keep you fueled during the workout, and a protein-rich meal afterward will encourage muscle repair and growth.

8.4. Periodically Revisit and Revise Your Plan

An effective routine should continually challenge you and facilitate progress towards your health and fitness goals. Once you become comfortable with your current routine, revisit your goals and evaluate your progress. Change can be brought in the form of new Pilates exercises, some adjustments in your workout schedule, or slight modifications in your nutrition plan.

Remember, the goal isn't to reach a destination, but to embark on a healthier lifestyle. A continuous fine-tuning of your nutrition and Pilates plan will only take you closer to achieving a perfect balance.

Exercising patience is as important as exercising your body. Adopting Pilates and pivoting into healthier eating patterns isn't a quick-fix, but a step-by-step transformation. Consistent effort will yield the results over time. Keep trusting the process, learn from lapses, and go a step further - towards a healthier, stronger you.

Chapter 9. Common Pitfalls and How to Avoid Them

There's no doubt that Pilates and proper nutrition can transform your physical and mental well-being. However, as beginners undertake this journey, they often face certain common pitfalls. Comprehending these challenges and knowing how to avoid them will magnify the benefits you reap, ensuring you remain motivated and committed.

9.1. Understanding The Misconceptions Around Pilates

Stemming from misinformation and lack of knowledge, misconceptions about Pilates are plentiful. Here are some common fallacies and the truths behind them:

1. 'Pilates is just for women:' This couldn't be further from the truth. Pilates was, in fact, developed by a man - Joseph Pilates - and is beneficial for everyone, regardless of gender.

2. 'Pilates is easy:' While it largely depends on approach and instructor, Pilates can be challenging even for seasoned athletes. This misconception can lead to disillusionment when individuals find it hard.

3. 'Pilates is similar to yoga:' Although both emphasize breath control and flexibility, Pilates focuses more on core strength, muscle toning, and body control.

To avoid these pitfalls, do thorough research and consult professionals before embarking on your Pilates journey.

9.2. Overlooking Nutrition's Role in Pilates

Just as a car needs fuel to run, your body needs the right nutrition to perform optimally. A key pitfall many face is ignoring nutrition when undertaking Pilates. The energy, endurance, and recovery needed for successful Pilates come from balanced nutrition. To counter this, incorporate a wholesome diet inclusive of:

- Lean proteins for muscle recovery

- Complex carbohydrates for sustained energy

- Healthy fats for essential fatty acids

- An abundance of fruits and vegetables for necessary vitamins and minerals

9.3. Neglecting Adequate Hydration

Hydration plays a crucial role in Pilates. Without optimal hydration, your muscles may cramp, your concentration may falter, and your performance could suffer. Aim to consume at least 8-10 glasses of water per day and increase intake during and after exercise to replace fluids lost through sweat.

9.4. Skipping Warm-ups and Cool-downs

Though tempting to dive straight into your routine, skipping warm-ups and cool-downs can lead to substantial issues, including injury and muscle aches. A proper warm-up prepares your body and mind for workout and a cool-down aids recovery, mitigating muscle soreness. Embrace them as integral parts of your routine.

9.5. Overdoing the Workout

It's easy to fall into the trap of over-exercising, especially with the surge of enthusiasm that comes with starting something new. Overworking your muscles can strain them and may lead to injury. It's essential to listen to your body and provide it adequate rest.

9.6. Ignoring Proper Form and Technique

Proper form is crucial to obtain maximum Pilates benefits. Regardless of how intense your workout is, if your form is incorrect, the results will likely be unsatisfactory and could lead to injuries. Always learn from a qualified professional, maintain control of your movements, and prioritize form over speed.

9.7. Unrealistic Expectations and Lack of Patience

As with any fitness regimen, results take time. Impatience and unrealistic expectations can not only lead to disappointment, but may also push you to overstrain yourself. Acknowledge that everybody is unique and that changes will occur at different rates for different individuals. The journey of fitness is lifelong, take it day by day.

These are some of the common pitfalls one must avoid on a Pilates journey. By being mindful of these potential obstacles, you're more likely to find the path to a healthier, energized, and balanced life smooth and rewarding. Remember, it's not just about the transformation of your body, but also of your mind and spirit. Embrace the journey with patience, commitment, and positivity, and the results will follow.

Chapter 10. Boosting Your Progress: Supplementary Exercises and Nutritional Tips

Progressing in Pilates and making the fitness routine more effective is as much about what you do on the mat as what you do off it. To maximize the benefits of your Pilates practice, it's essential to incorporate supportive exercises into your routine and to make mindful nutritional choices.

10.1. Supplementary Exercises

The role of supplementary exercises in Pilates cannot be overstated. They help to reinforce the gains made through the primary workout by strengthening the core muscles, increasing overall body strength, and enhancing flexibility.

Anchor exercises in Pilates consist of concentrating on key muscle groups. Doing these supplementary exercises regularly can give the usual Pilates workout a significant boost.

Table 1. Top Supplementary Exercises

Exercise	Description	Benefit
Planks	Holding a position similar to a push-up, but with elbows bent and resting on your forearms.	Enhances core stability, and strengthens shoulders and arm muscles.

Exercise	Description	Benefit
Squats	Standing with feet hip-width apart, bend knees and lower your body as far as you can.	Strengthens lower body, enhances flexibility, and improves posture.
Push-ups	Beginning in a high plank position, lower your body until your chest nearly touches the floor, then push your body back up.	Works upper body and core.
Bridges	Lying on your back with knees bent and feet flat on the floor, raise your hips off the floor.	Strengthens glutes and hamstrings, and opens up hip flexors.
Bicycle crunches	Lying flat on your back, bring one knee and the opposite elbow together in a slow and controlled manner, alternating sides.	Strengthens abdominal muscles and improves coordination.

In order to see continuous improvement, it is important to keep rotating and updating these exercises at regular intervals. Changing the routine not only helps address all muscle groups but also helps maintain interest and motivation.

10.2. Nutritional Tips

Implementing a healthy, balanced diet is equally as important in achieving fitness goals. Here are some practical and dietitian-approved nutritional tips for those engaging in a Pilates routine.

Table 2. Nutritional Tips for Improved Fitness

Tip	Description
Hydrate	Regular and adequate water intake is crucial not only for overall health but also for muscle function and recovery after workouts.
Balanced meals	Each meal should include a balance of lean protein (for muscle repair), complex carbohydrates (for energy), and healthy fats (for satiety).
Pre-workout snacks	A combination of protein and carbohydrates before workout sessions can provide sustained energy.
Post-workout recovery food	A post-Pilates meal or snack that includes both protein and carbohydrates can aid muscle recovery and replenishment of energy stores.
Regular meals	Keeping a regular eating schedule helps to maintain stable energy levels throughout the day.

Remember, the relationship between diet and exercise is symbiotic. They work together to create a healthy body and mind. By integrating these nutritional tips into your daily routine, you're setting yourself up for success in your Pilates practice.

10.3. Real-Life Success Stories

To bring these tips to life, we spoke to individuals who have enhanced their Pilates practice through supplementary exercises and improved nutrition.

Kyle, a 35-year-old engineer, shared that incorporating supplementary exercises like push-ups and squats into his routine not only improved his strength but also his performance in Pilates. Simultaneously, he made changes to his diet, such as increasing protein intake and maintaining a regular eating schedule. These changes not only boosted his energy levels but also helped him recover faster after workouts.

Another success story is Erica, a 42-year-old teacher and mother of two. Despite having a hectic schedule, Erica managed to regularly fit in quick supplementary exercises. She also started making conscious food choices, ensuring well-balanced meals for herself and her family. Within a few months, Erica noticed significant improvements in her strength, flexibility, and overall health.

While everyone's journey is unique, the underlying message is clear: a balanced approach that includes Pilates, supplementary exercises, and mindful eating is a powerful formula for achieving health and fitness goals.

Stay motivated, keeping in mind that transformation is a process, not a single event. The path to a stronger and healthier self is a marathon, not a sprint. By incorporating Pilates into your life, alongside these supplementary exercises and nutritional tips, you are laying the foundation for a healthier, more fulfilling and balanced lifestyle.

Chapter 11. Manifesting Wellness: Sustaining Your Pilates Habit Beyond The Mat

Well-balanced wellness goes beyond the confines of the Pilates studio. It spills over into every aspect of our daily lives, immersing us in a holistic approach to health. Achieving this wellness does not occur overnight but is a continued practice, an embodiment of the very essence of Pilates itself - intentional, controlled movements leading to powerful transformations.

11.1. The Art of Incorporation

A common misconception about Pilates is that it is constrained to the mat or reformer. However, Joseph Pilates meant for the techniques and principles to transcend the physical exercises and become a part of your daily living. Herein lies the real power of Pilates.

Think about the profound yet straightforward principle of 'Control.' This principle underscores the importance of being mindful about every movement - each extension, each contraction. Now take this principle off the mat, and apply it to your eating habits. Imagine being more conscious of what you're eating, why you're eating it, and how it makes you feel. Or consider the principle of 'Flow,' which promotes fluidity and grace in movement, and applying it to how you navigate your daily life and tasks.

These real-life applications of Pilates principles foster not only physical health, but they also promote mental and emotional well-being by enabling mindfulness, discipline, and a more profound sense of control over our own lives.

11.2. The Power of Nutritional Balance

Nutrition is a vital aspect that directly influences our energy levels, our physiology, and subsequently, our Pilates performance. From consuming enough proteins for muscle repair and recovery to healthy fats for long-lasting energy, each element of our diet plays a crucial role. Becoming mindful of good nutrition, understanding what our body needs, and responding to it accurately can profoundly impact our Pilates practice and overall health.

Take, for example, hydration, a vital yet often neglected component of nutrition. Maintaining internal hydration aids in muscle elasticity and joint lubrication, directly affecting flexibility and overall physical performance. By making a conscious effort to hydrate consistently, we not only help our bodies perform better during Pilates but also promote healthier skin, better digestion, and an overall sense of well-being.

11.3. Insights into Meal Planning and Prepping

For many, the concept of 'health eating' can be overwhelming, with numerous dietary theories and countless 'superfoods.' A significant challenge is often translating this information into practical, everyday eating habits. The first step in this journey is to understand further and respect your body's unique nutritional requirements and respond to its cues.

Meal planning and meal prepping can be transformational methods. Evaluating your week ahead, identifying potential challenges or busy days, and planning your meals and snacks can drastically reduce last-minute unhealthier food choices. Preparation could also involve portioning out your meals and snacks for each day, which works beautifully with the Pilates principle of 'Precision.'

11.4. The Role of Rest

Rest, often the most undervalued aspect of health, is paramount to balance and wellness. It impacts not just physical recovery and growth, but mental wellness too. Just as 'Balance' is key in Pilates - in every pose, every sequence - it holds in life as well. By balancing active moments with restful ones, we align ourselves more closely with wellness.

11.5. A Journey, Not a Destination

As Joseph Pilates once said, "Patience and persistence are vital qualities in the ultimate successful accomplishment of any worthwhile endeavor." Manifesting wellness through Pilates beyond the mat is a journey, not a destination. It's a personal voyage of discovering balance, finding harmony, and nurturing strength, both within and without.

In a nutshell, the road to wellness does not end after a fulfilling Pilates session. It continues with us as we navigate our everyday lives, making mindful choices that encapsulate the core of Pilates principles. It thrives on the fusion of conscious movement with conscious nutrition - a beautiful synergy aimed at fueling the body, healing the mind, and nourishing the soul. Remember, every moment is an opportunity to make a more balanced choice, a chance to bring the power of Pilates into our lives. So, let's embrace it and embark on this transformational journey together.